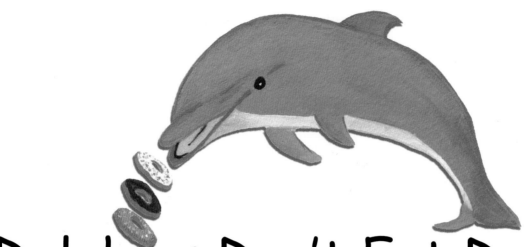

Dolphins Don't Eat Donuts

Written and Illustrated by Julianne Stokes

Published in Snowmass Village, Colorado.
Printed in China.
ISBN: 978-0-692-13082-7
Library of Congress Control Number: 2018907796

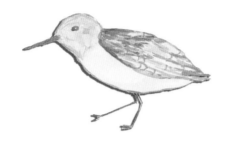

To Piper who loves to dance and prance like a little sandpiper.

Dolphins don't eat donuts.

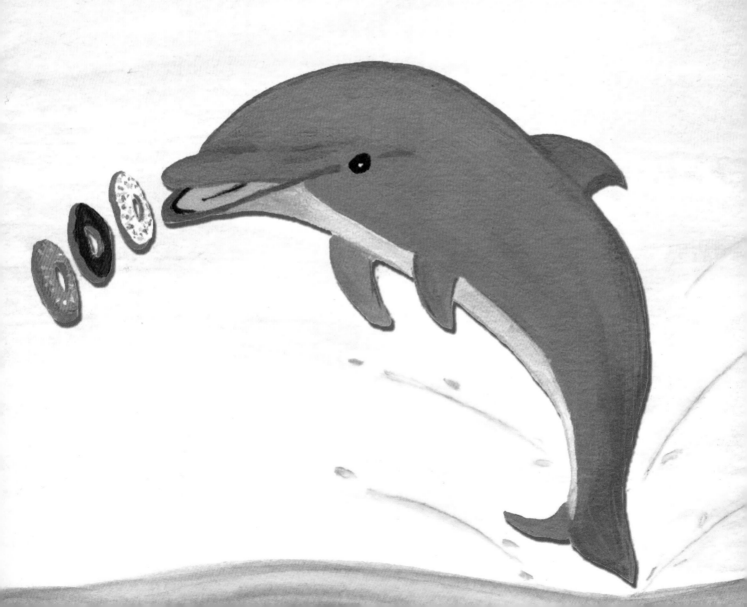

Dogs don't eat candy.

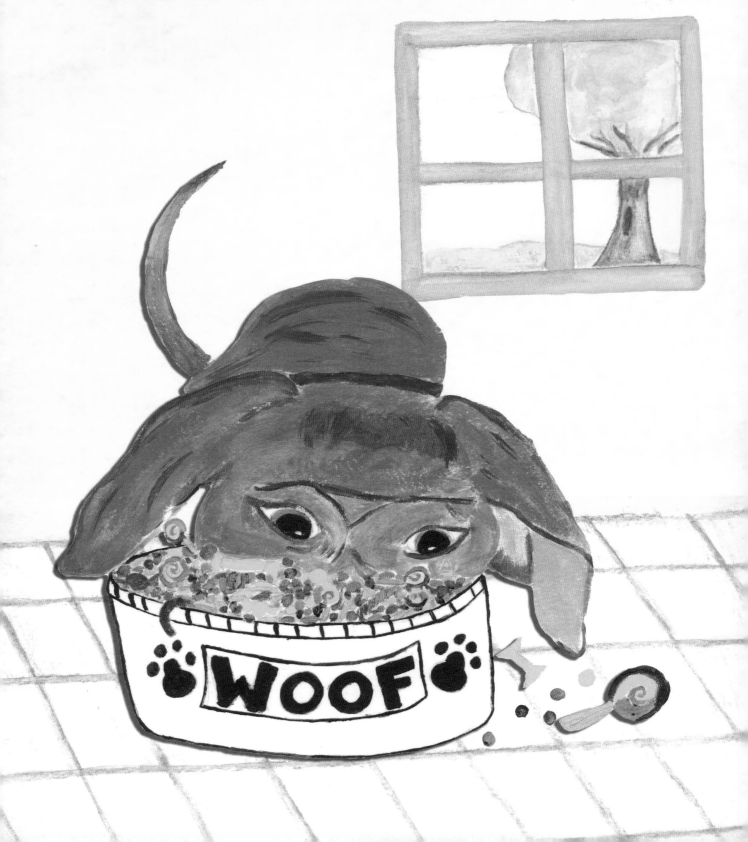

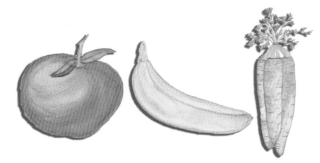

Learning from our animal friends might be kind of handy!

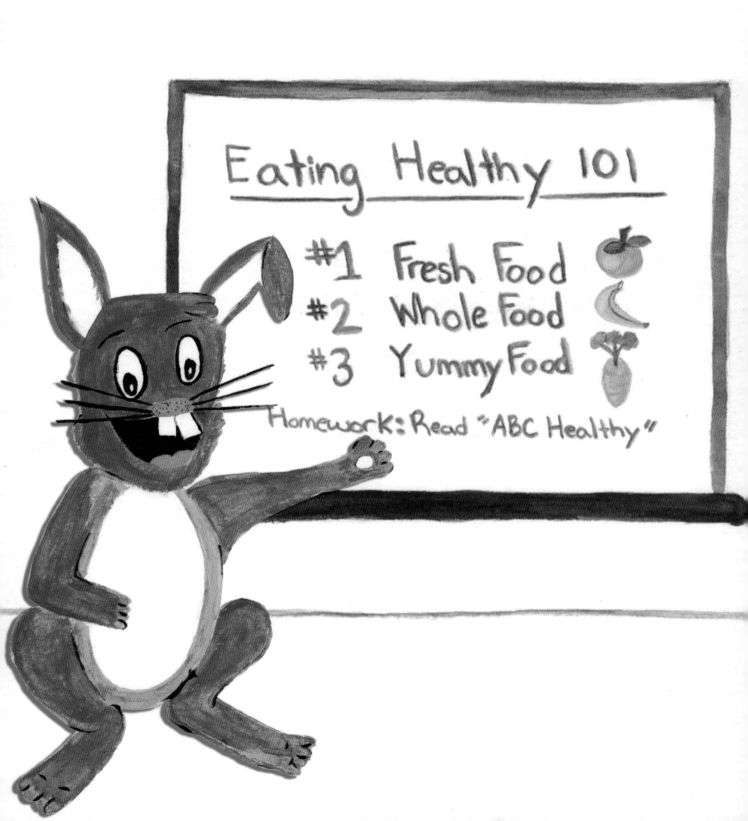

Bears eat fish.

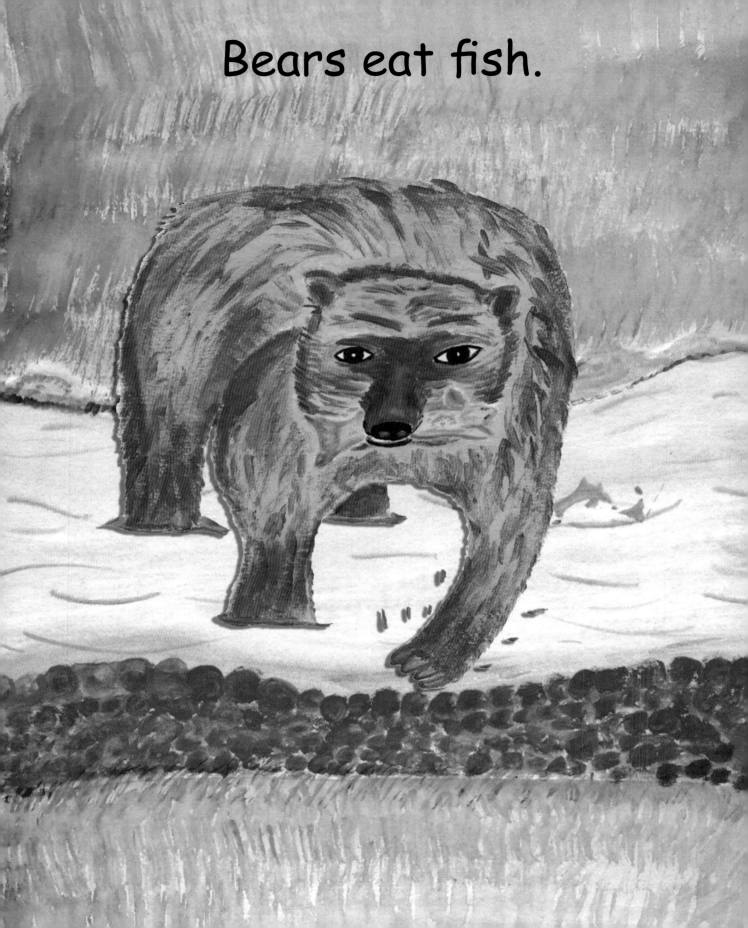

Birds eat berries.

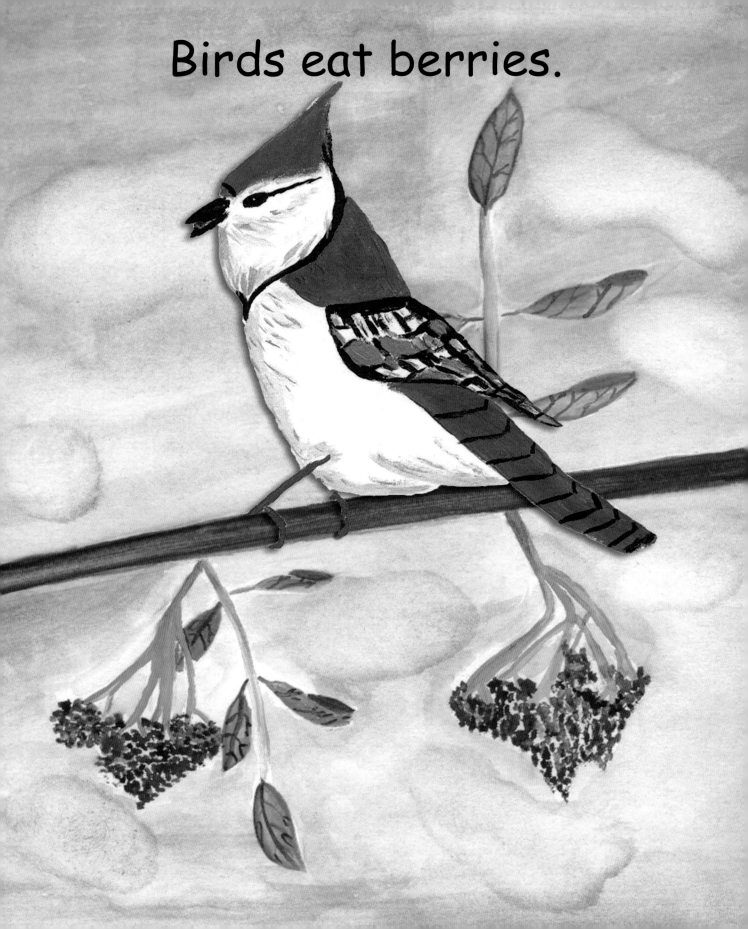

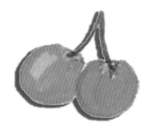

If you are looking for a healthy treat grab some delicious cherries!

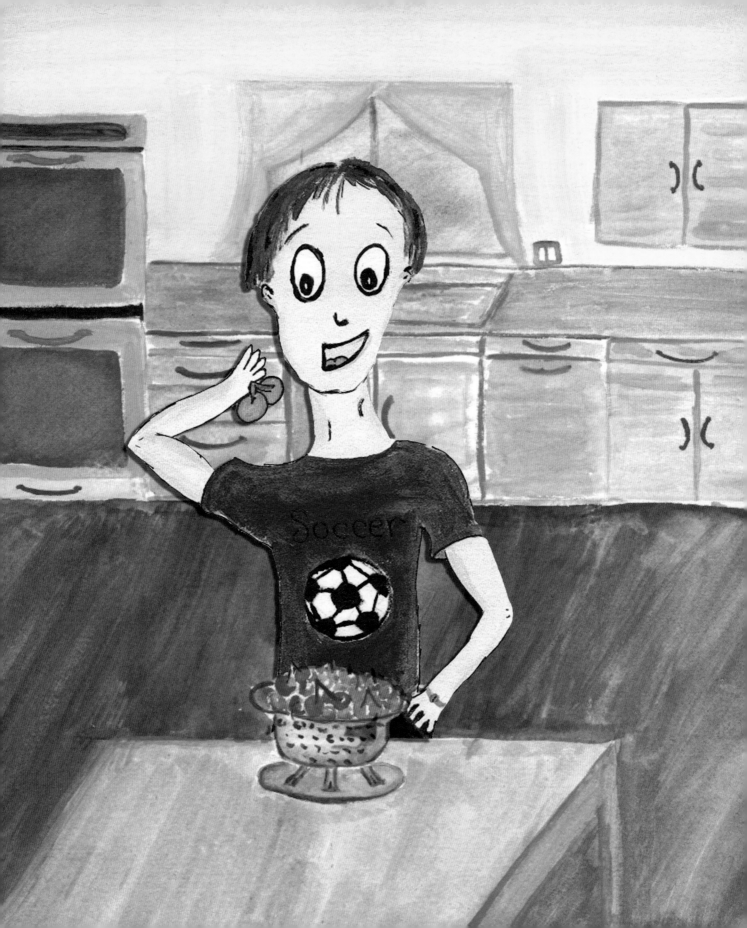

Turtles don't eat jelly rolls.

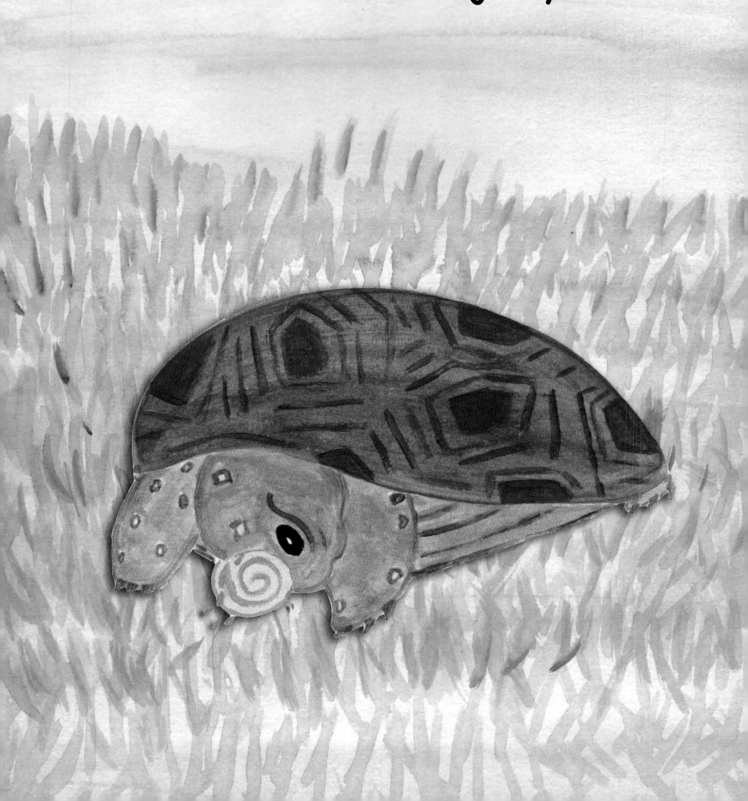

Cows don't eat lollypops.

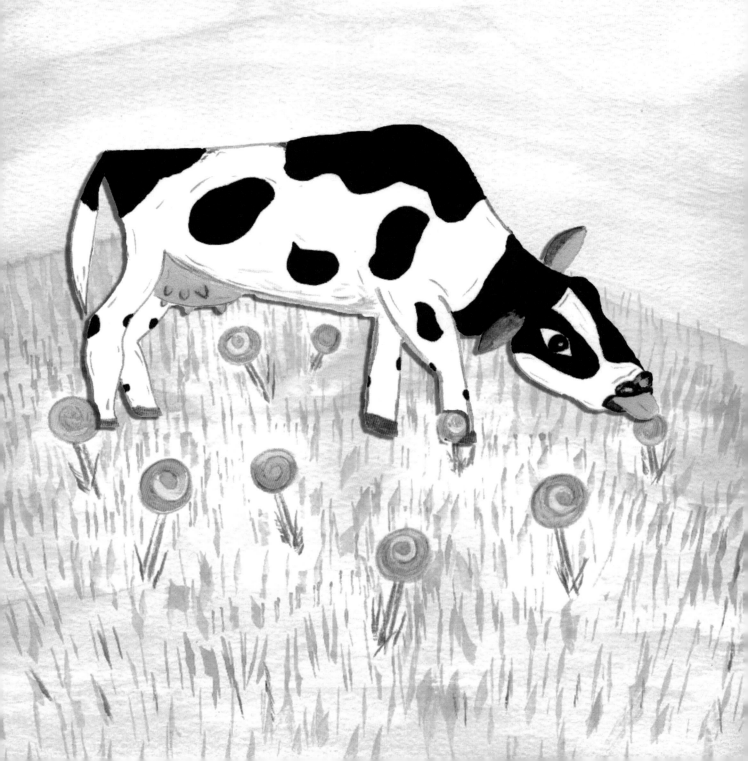

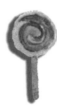

If you go to a farm you will never see candy crops!

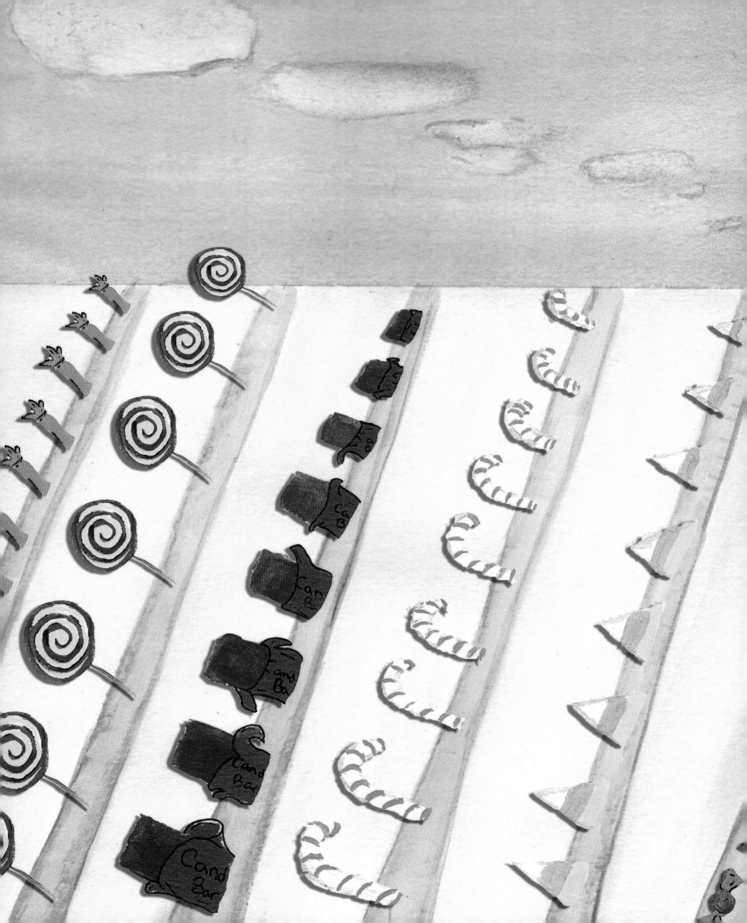

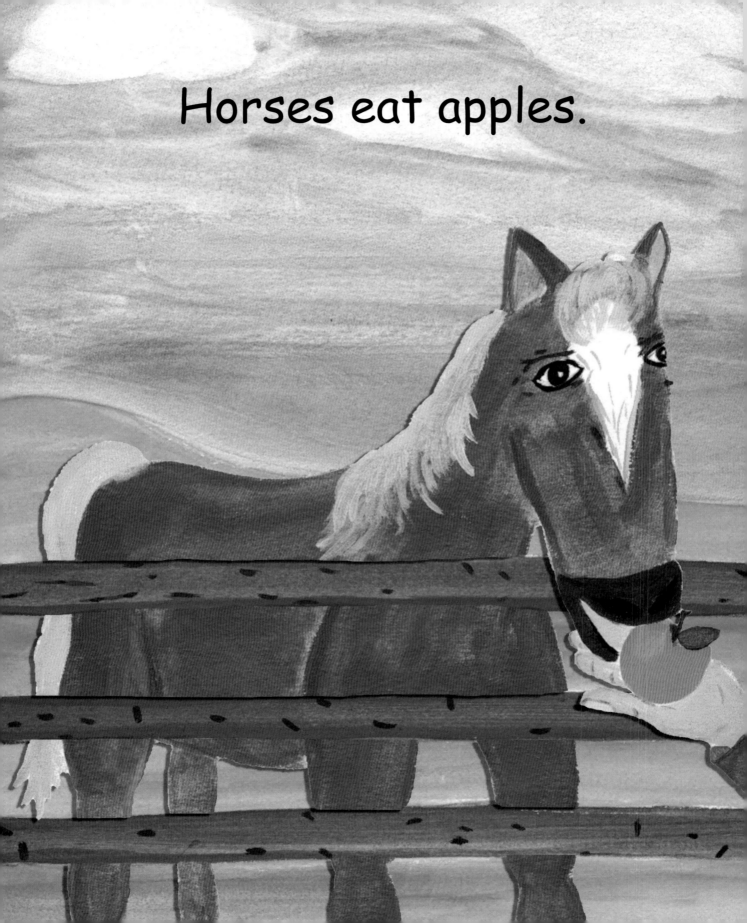

Horses eat apples.

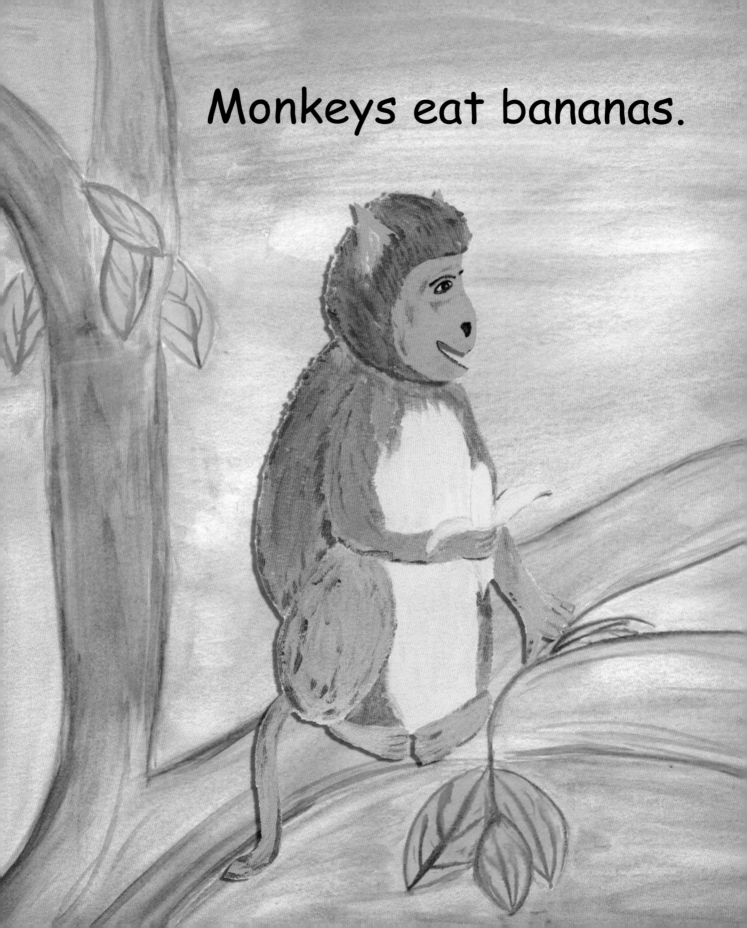

Monkeys eat bananas.

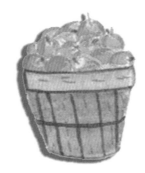

Put some fruit in a basket or simply use bandanas!

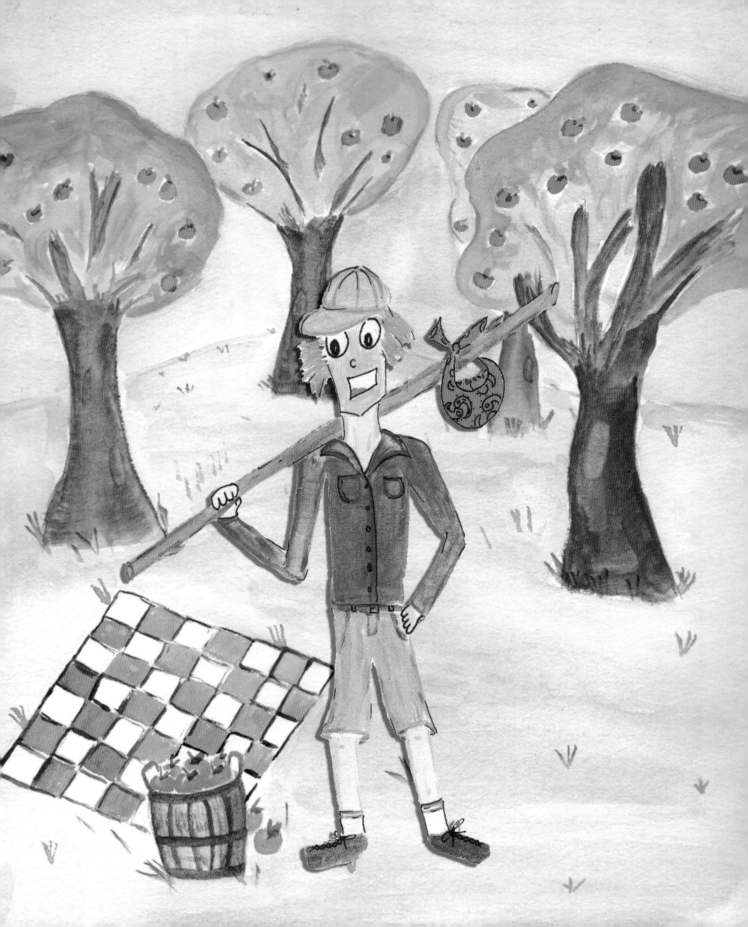

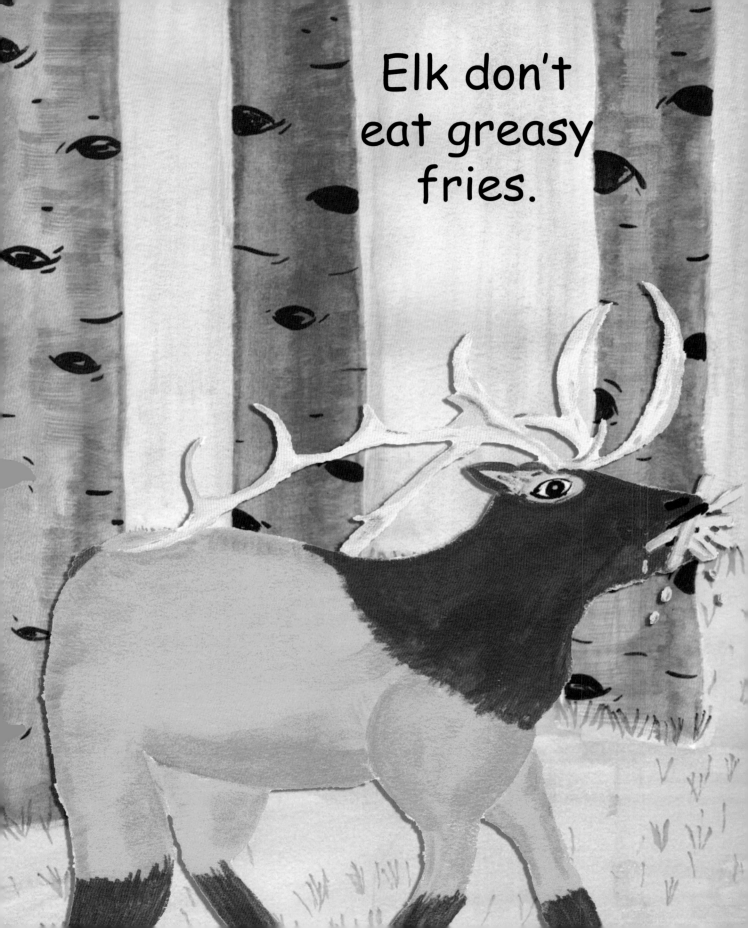

Foxes don't eat potato chips.

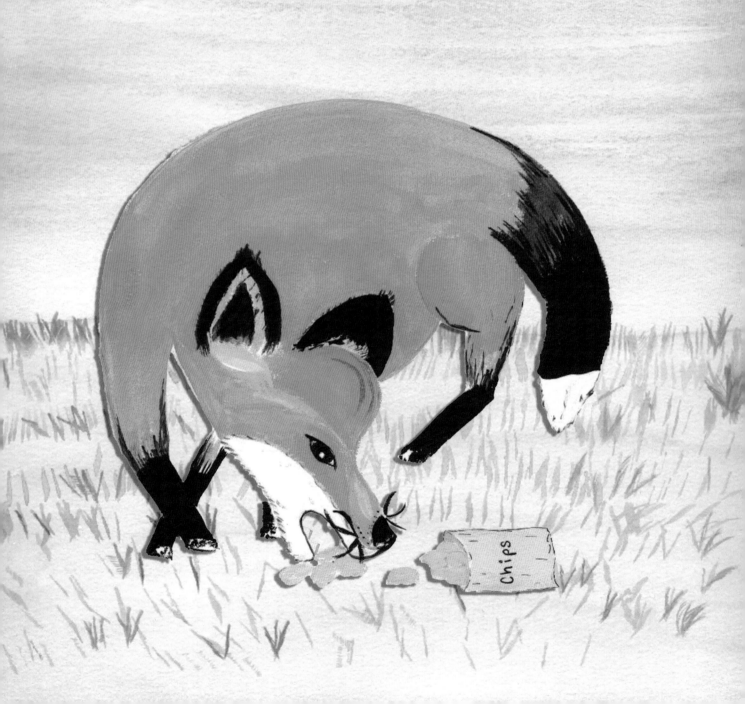

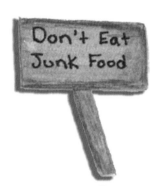

If these animals talked they would give you healthy tips!

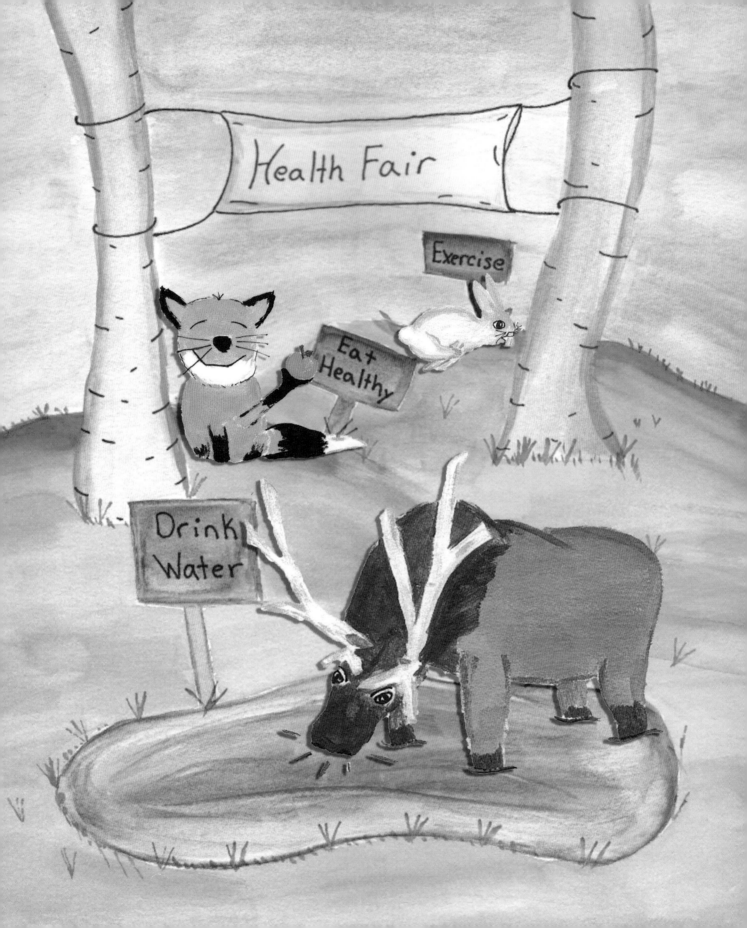

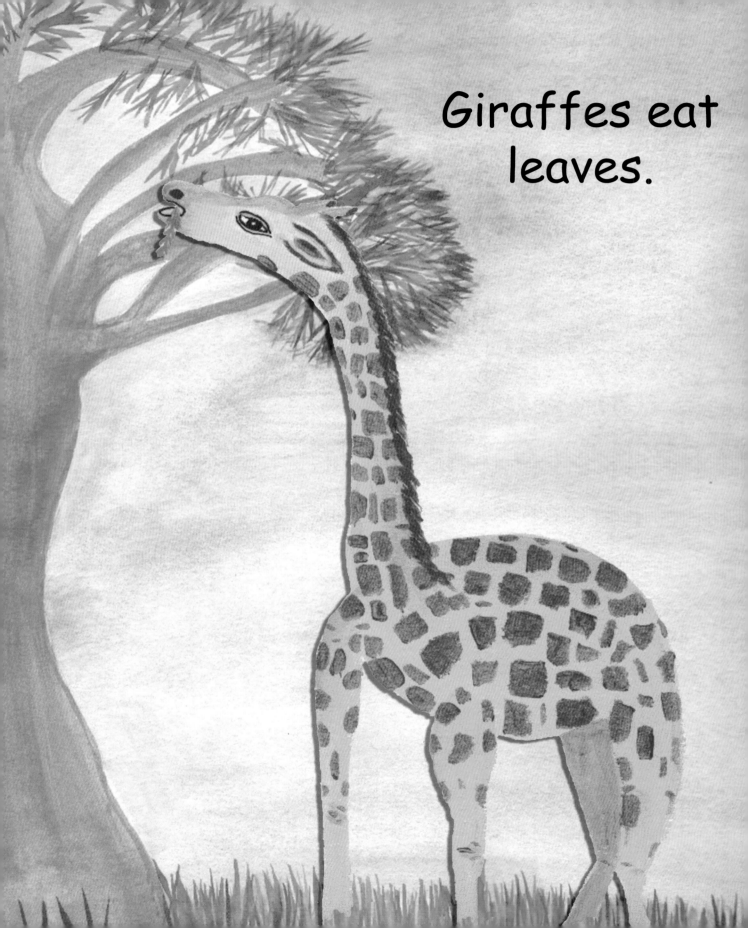

Giraffes eat leaves.

Pandas eat bamboo.

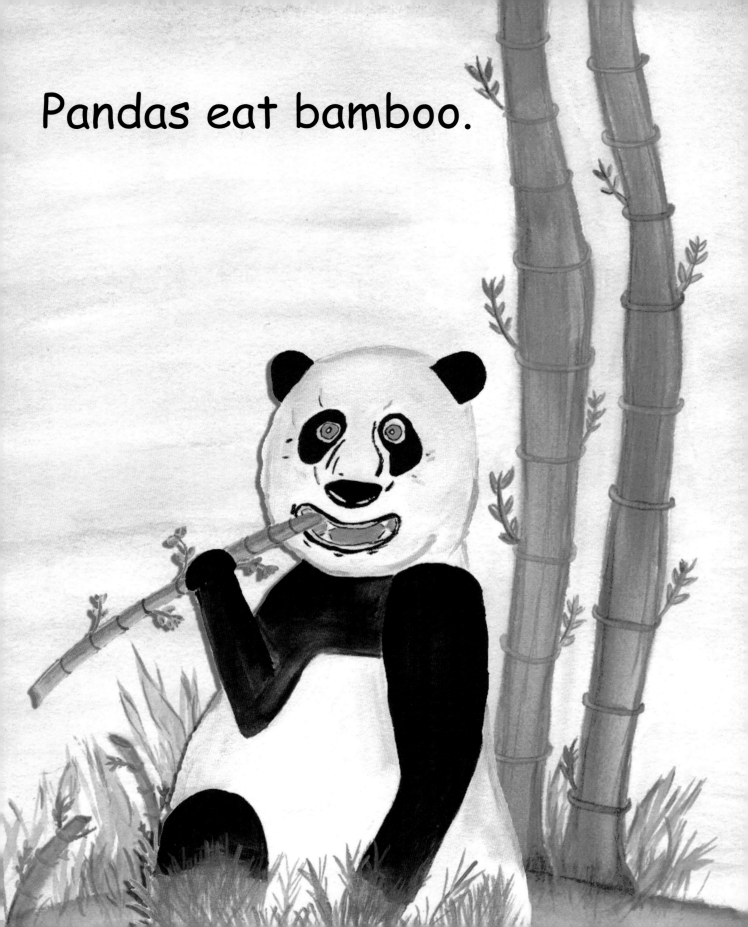

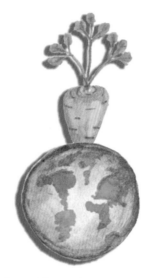

Eating food from the earth is the ultimate thing to do!

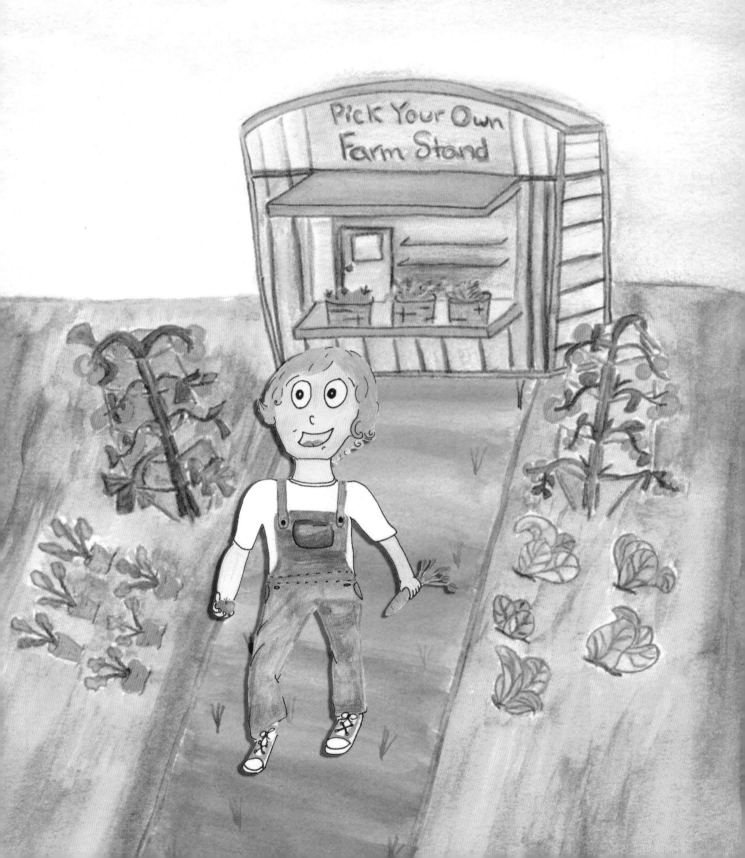

It is simple you see, our animal friends are naturally healthy. So put away the candy corn and have a sweet potato. Give healthy treats a try and you will be strong as a tornado!

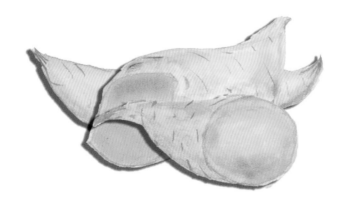

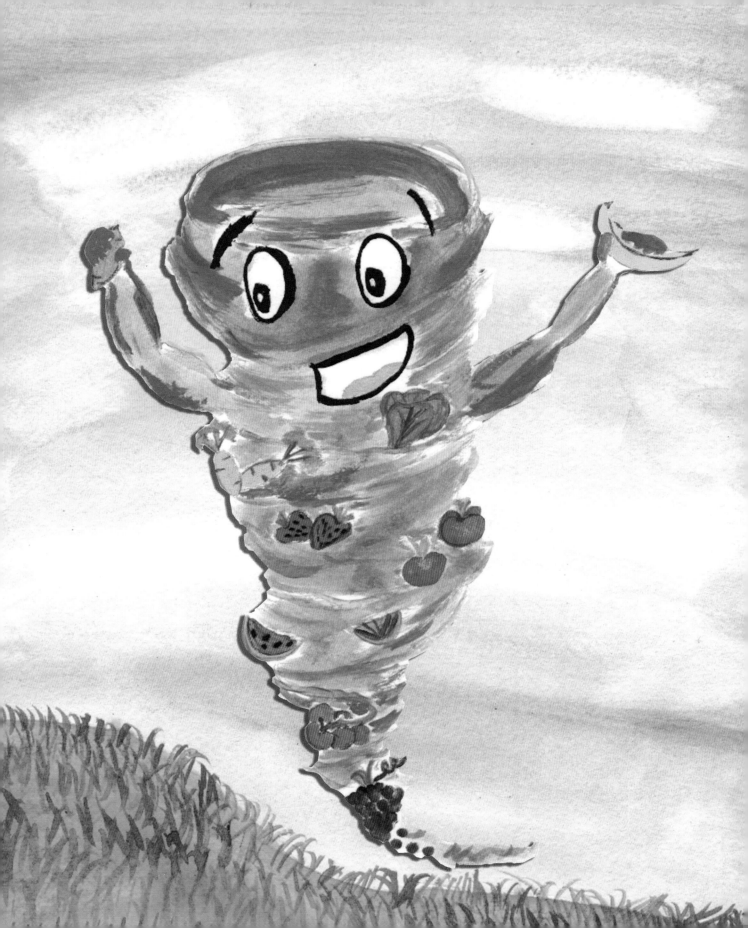

Thank you to Owen who is strong as a tornado!

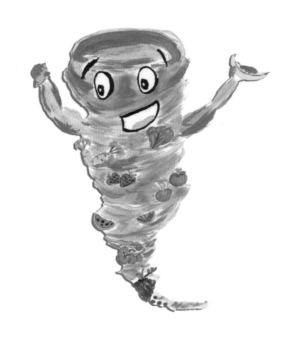